THE MENOPAUSE MANIFESTO DIET COOKBOOK

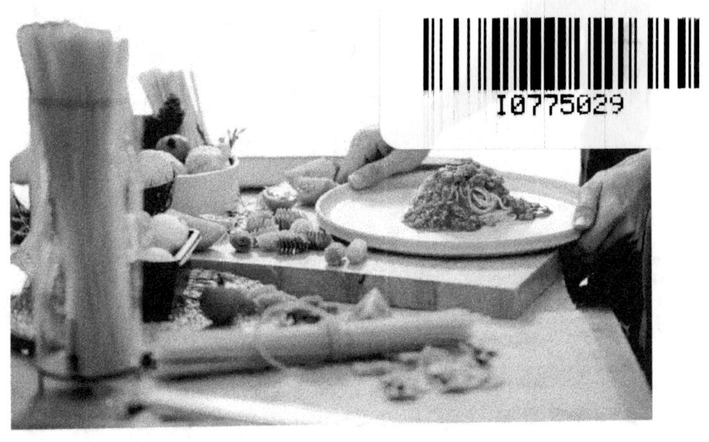

A comprehensive guide in creating and managing hormones, physical and emotional health during the change

ERIN P. WALKER

Copyright © 2023 by Erin P. Walker

Table of contents

Introduction

In the quiet town of Willowbrook, Evelyn, a woman in her early fifties, grappled with the unwelcome companionship of menopausal symptoms. Sleepless nights, sudden hot flashes, and an inexplicable weight gain seemed to have taken residence in her life. Feeling determined to regain control, Evelyn wandered into the local bookstore one afternoon, searching for a solution amidst the shelves of wisdom.

There, she stumbled upon a promising guide. Intrigued, Evelyn decided to give it a chance. Little did she know that within the pages of this book lay the keys to a transformative journey.

As Evelyn immersed herself in the contents, she discovered a wealth of knowledge about the science behind menopause and practical strategies for managing its effects through nutrition and lifestyle changes. The guide wasn't just a manual; it was a compassionate guide that spoke directly to her struggles and offered a roadmap to navigate this transitional phase of life.

Evelyn began incorporating the guide's recommendations into her daily routine. Processed snacks made way for nourishing fruits and vegetables, and her meals became a colourful array of superfoods known to alleviate menopausal symptoms. The guide's carefully crafted meal plans and recipes became her allies, turning her kitchen into a sanctuary of health.

What surprised Evelyn the most was the emphasis on exercise tailored for women undergoing menopause. The guide introduced her to a range of activities that not only addressed the changes in her body but also brought a renewed sense of joy and energy to her life. From brisk morning walks to evening yoga sessions, Evelyn discovered a love for movement that she hadn't known before.

Weeks passed, and Evelyn began to witness remarkable changes. The frequency of hot flashes diminished, her sleep improved, and the stubborn weight started to dissipate. The guide had become her trusted companion, guiding her through the challenges with a blend of science, practicality, and empathy.

Beyond the physical transformations, the guide also delved into the emotional aspects of menopause. Evelyn found solace in its chapters on stress management and emotional eating. The strategies provided became invaluable tools, helping her navigate the emotional ups and downs that often accompanied hormonal fluctuations.

Word of Evelyn's positive journey spread throughout Willowbrook, and soon, other women in the town turned to similar guides for guidance. The bookstore shelves quickly emptied, creating a sense of shared camaraderie among the women as they embarked on this journey together.

Evelyn's story became a beacon of inspiration not only for her fellow townspeople but for women far and wide facing the challenges of menopause. What started as a simple bookstore discovery became a powerful agent of change, as women like Evelyn embraced the wisdom of the guide and forged a path toward a healthier, more vibrant life beyond menopause.

A cookbook tailored to support your menopause journey can play a crucial role in managing the physical and emotional changes associated with this life stage. Here's a comprehensive explanation of how a Menopause Manifesto Diet Cookbook can be a valuable resource:

1. Nutrient Optimization:

- The cookbook provides recipes specifically designed to address the nutritional needs of women going through menopause. It focuses on incorporating foods rich in essential nutrients like calcium, vitamin D, omega-3 fatty acids, and phytoestrogens, which can help alleviate common menopausal symptoms.

2. Hormone-Balancing Ingredients:

   - Many recipes in the cookbook include ingredients known for their hormone-balancing properties. For instance, certain herbs, spices, and plant-based foods can contribute to hormonal equilibrium, helping to manage mood swings, hot flashes, and other hormonal fluctuations.

3. Weight Management and Metabolism:

   - Menopause often brings about changes in metabolism and weight distribution. The cookbook offers recipes that support a healthy weight through a balanced mix of lean proteins, whole grains, and fibre-rich fruits and vegetables. These recipes can help women maintain a healthy weight during and after menopause.

4. Energy and Vitality:

   - Menopausal symptoms, such as fatigue and decreased energy levels, can impact daily life. The cookbook emphasises recipes that are rich in nutrients, providing sustained energy throughout the day. Balanced meals and snacks help combat energy slumps and promote overall vitality.

5. Bone Health and Calcium Intake:

   - Menopausal women are often at an increased risk of bone density loss. The cookbook includes recipes with ingredients high in calcium and vitamin D, crucial for maintaining bone health. This supports women in minimising the risk of osteoporosis and related issues.

6. Emotional Well-being:

- The cookbook acknowledges the emotional challenges that can accompany menopause. It includes recipes with ingredients known to support mood and emotional well-being. For example, certain foods contain compounds that can positively impact serotonin levels, promoting a sense of happiness and calm.

7. Meal Planning and Convenience:

- Menopausal women often face time constraints and may find it challenging to plan nutritious meals. The cookbook offers practical meal planning tips, easy-to-follow recipes, and suggestions for batch cooking. This makes it more convenient for women to maintain a healthy diet despite a busy lifestyle.

8. Social and Lifestyle Integration:

- Menopause can sometimes impact social activities and dietary choices. The cookbook provides guidance on making healthy choices when dining out, hosting gatherings, or attending social events. It empowers women to enjoy food-related aspects of life while still adhering to their menopause-friendly dietary goals.

9. Long-Term Lifestyle Adoption:

- The cookbook encourages women to view their menopause diet as a sustainable and enjoyable lifestyle rather than a short-term fix. By providing a variety of flavorful recipes and emphasising a balanced approach, the cookbook supports women in making lasting changes that contribute to overall health and well-being.

In summary, a Menopause Manifesto Diet Cookbook serves as a comprehensive guide, offering not just recipes but a holistic approach to nutrition tailored to the unique needs and challenges of menopausal women. It empowers women to take control of their health through delicious and nutritious meals, promoting a positive and fulfilling menopause journey.

Understanding the Link Between Nutrition and Menopause

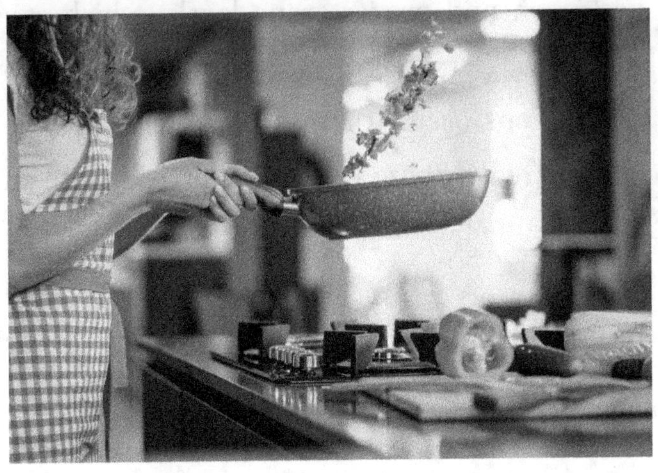

Understanding the link between nutrition and menopause is crucial for women navigating this significant life stage. The hormonal changes that accompany menopause can have profound effects on a woman's body, impacting various aspects of her health and well-being. Nutrition plays a pivotal role in mitigating the symptoms and promoting overall health during and after menopause. Here's a comprehensive exploration of the link between nutrition and menopause:

1. Hormonal Changes and Metabolism:

- Menopause is marked by a decline in oestrogen and progesterone levels, which can influence metabolism. As hormonal fluctuations occur, there is a tendency for the body to redistribute weight, often leading to an increase in abdominal fat. Proper nutrition can help manage these changes by supporting a healthy metabolism through balanced meals and portion control.

2. Bone Health and Calcium Requirements:

- Oestrogen plays a crucial role in maintaining bone density, and its decline during menopause can lead to an increased risk of osteoporosis. Adequate calcium intake becomes essential. Nutrition during menopause focuses on incorporating foods rich in calcium, such as dairy products, leafy green vegetables, and fortified foods, to support bone health.

3. Cardiovascular Health:

- Menopausal women face an increased risk of cardiovascular issues. Nutrition strategies include adopting a heart-healthy diet that is low in saturated fats, trans fats, and cholesterol. Emphasis is placed on incorporating omega-3 fatty acids, found in fatty fish, flaxseeds, and walnuts, to support cardiovascular health.

4. Blood Sugar Management:

- Hormonal changes can also influence insulin sensitivity, impacting blood sugar levels. A balanced diet with a focus on complex carbohydrates, fibre-rich foods, and lean proteins helps regulate blood sugar levels. This approach can be instrumental in preventing or managing conditions such as insulin resistance and type 2 diabetes.

5. Mood and Emotional Well-being:

- Menopause can be accompanied by mood swings, irritability, and anxiety. Nutrition plays a role in supporting emotional well-being by including foods that contribute to the production of neurotransmitters like serotonin. Whole grains, fruits, and vegetables contain nutrients that support a positive mood.

6. Hormone-Balancing Foods:

   - Certain foods, known as phytoestrogens, have compounds that mimic the effects of oestrogen in the body. Soy products, flaxseeds, and legumes are examples of foods that can potentially help balance hormonal fluctuations during menopause.

7. Managing Menopausal Symptoms:

   - Nutrition can be tailored to manage specific menopausal symptoms. For instance, incorporating foods rich in phytoestrogens may help alleviate hot flashes. Foods with anti-inflammatory properties, such as fatty fish and fruits rich in antioxidants, can contribute to managing joint pain and inflammation.

8. Weight Management:

   - Menopausal women may experience changes in body composition and weight distribution. Nutrition strategies focus on maintaining a healthy weight through a balanced diet that includes lean proteins, whole grains, and plenty of fruits and vegetables. Portion control and mindful eating are emphasised to prevent unwanted weight gain.

9. Importance of Micronutrients:

   - Micronutrients like vitamins and minerals become particularly important during menopause. Ensuring an adequate intake of vitamins D and E, calcium, magnesium, and other essential nutrients is vital for overall health, immune function, and bone strength.

10. Long-Term Lifestyle Considerations:

   - Beyond managing immediate symptoms, nutrition during menopause is framed as a long-term lifestyle consideration. Adopting a well-rounded and sustainable approach to eating ensures that women not only navigate the challenges of menopause but also promote overall health and well-being in the years that follow.

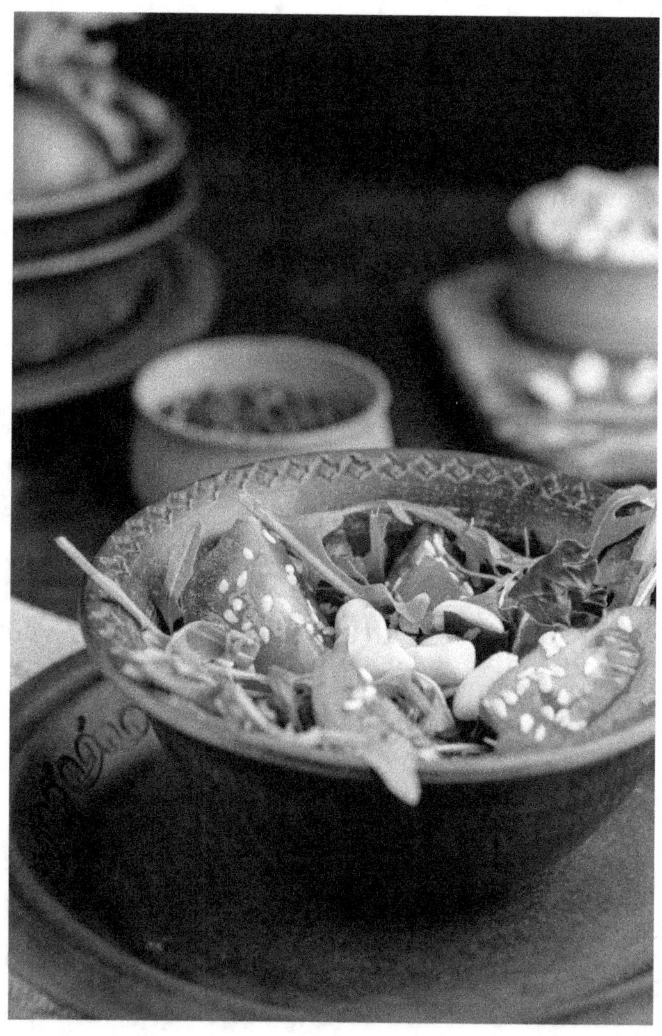

Chapter 1

Overview of Menopausal Changes

The menopausal transition is a natural phase in a woman's life, typically occurring in her late 40s or early 50s, although the exact timing can vary. During this period, the ovaries gradually reduce their production of oestrogen and progesterone, leading to a cessation of menstrual cycles and a range of hormonal changes. Understanding the overview of menopausal changes is essential for women navigating this significant life stage.

Menopausal changes are primarily driven by hormonal fluctuations. As oestrogen levels decline, women may experience various physical and emotional shifts. Common symptoms include hot flashes, night sweats, vaginal dryness, and changes in sleep patterns. The decline in oestrogen can also contribute to bone density loss, potentially increasing the risk of osteoporosis.

Weight management becomes a concern for many women during menopause. Metabolism tends to slow down, and there may be a redistribution of body fat, often leading to an increase in abdominal fat. These changes can pose challenges to maintaining a healthy weight and body composition.

Menopause can also impact cardiovascular health. Changes in hormone levels may contribute to an increase in cholesterol levels and a higher risk of heart disease. It becomes crucial for women to focus on heart-healthy nutrition and lifestyle habits during this phase.

Emotionally, menopause can bring about mood swings, irritability, and increased susceptibility to stress and anxiety. The hormonal fluctuations, coupled with life changes associated with ageing, can contribute to these emotional shifts. Maintaining emotional well-being becomes an integral aspect of navigating menopausal changes.

Bone health is another significant consideration during menopause. With the decline in oestrogen, women become more susceptible to bone density loss, leading to an increased risk of fractures and osteoporosis. Adequate calcium intake and weight-bearing exercises are essential for preserving bone health.

Understanding the overview of menopausal changes is not just about recognizing the physical symptoms but also acknowledging the individuality of the menopausal experience. Each woman may experience menopause differently, with some navigating it smoothly, while others may face more pronounced challenges. This awareness underscores the importance of tailored approaches to nutrition, exercise, and emotional well-being during this transitional phase.

Navigating this phase requires a holistic understanding of these changes, empowering women to adopt strategies that support their unique journey through menopause.

Creating a Balanced Menopause-Friendly Diet

Menopause brings many changes to a woman's body, including potential weight gain, hot flashes, sleep disturbances, and mood swings. While hormone therapy can help alleviate some of these symptoms, adjusting your diet is another effective way to manage menopause. Here are some tips for creating a nutritious, balanced diet to help you thrive during this transition:

Focus on Whole Foods

Aim to get most of your nutrition from unprocessed "real" foods like fruits, vegetables, whole grains, lean proteins, nuts and seeds. These foods are packed with vitamins, minerals and fibre that can help stabilise hormones and energy levels. Limit refined carbs, added sugars and processed foods which can cause spikes and crashes in blood sugar.

Power Up with Protein

Protein is essential for building and repairing cells and muscles. Good sources include eggs, poultry, fish, beans, lentils, nuts and seeds. Aim for 20-30 grams of protein per meal to help you feel satisfied. This can help prevent weight gain and loss of muscle mass during menopause.

Include Phytoestrogen Foods

Phytoestrogens are plant compounds that mimic weak oestrogen activity in the body. Foods like flaxseeds, soy, nuts, oats and legumes contain phytoestrogens that may help relieve hot flashes, night sweats and other symptoms. Try adding them to your diet to see if they provide relief.

Stock Up on Calcium and Vitamin D

Menopause increases your risk of osteoporosis and bone fractures. Boost your calcium intake with milk, yoghurt, cheese, leafy greens, sardines and supplements if needed. Get sufficient Vitamin D from eggs, salmon, tuna, mushrooms and safe sun exposure for absorption. Weight bearing exercises are also key for bone health.

Stay Hydrated

Hormone changes can cause water retention and bloating. Counteract this by drinking plenty of water, herbal tea and fluids daily. Limit alcohol and sugary or caffeinated drinks which can exacerbate symptoms like hot flashes. Proper hydration promotes general health too.

Listen to Your Body

There is no one-size-fits-all menopause diet. Pay attention to how different foods affect your energy, mood, weight and symptoms. Tailor your diet accordingly to optimise your nutrition and wellbeing during this transition.

Creating a nutritious, balanced diet can make a big difference when it comes to managing menopausal symptoms gracefully. Focus on whole foods, proper hydration, phytoestrogens and nutrients for bone health. Listen to your body's needs and adjust your eating habits to thrive during menopause and beyond.

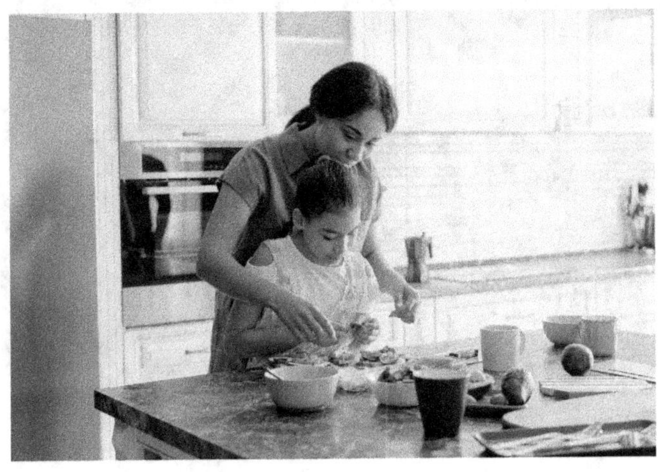

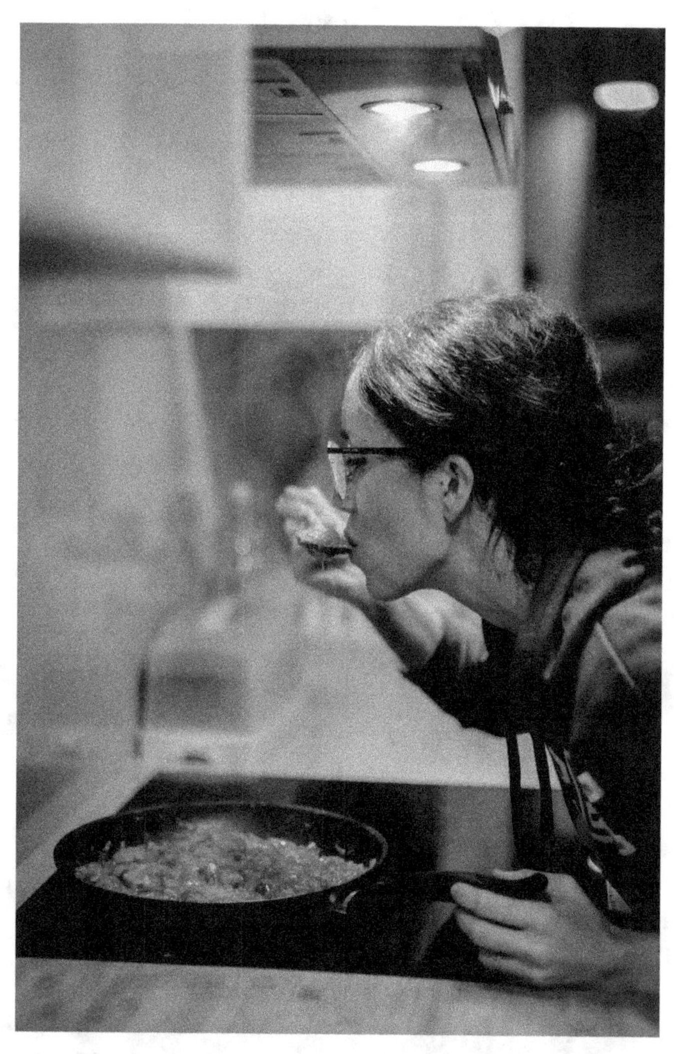

Chapter 2

Essential Pantry Staples

Healthy Fats

- Extra virgin olive oil - Contains antioxidants and phytoestrogens. Use for cooking, dressings and marinades.

- Avocados - Great source of monounsaturated fats. Eat them fresh or use avocado oil for cooking.

- Nuts and seeds - Packed with healthy fats, protein and minerals. Keep varieties like almonds, walnuts, sunflower seeds on hand.

- Fatty fish - Salmon, mackerel and sardines are rich in anti-inflammatory omega-3s. Roast, grill or eat canned food.

Protein Sources

- Eggs - A superfood packed with high-quality protein, vitamins and antioxidants like choline.

- Beans and legumes - Kidney beans, chickpeas, lentils provide plant-based protein, fibre and phytoestrogens.

- Tofu and tempeh - Soy-based proteins offer isoflavones that may help relieve hot flashes.

- Bone broth - Sip this to provide collagen, amino acids and minerals for bone and joint health.

Whole Grains

- Oats - Great source of soluble fibre to help control cholesterol and blood sugar levels.

- Quinoa - Highly nutritious grain with protein and antioxidants. Use in place of rice or oats.

- Brown rice - Has more fibre than white rice and contains magnesium for bones and energy.

- Whole grain bread - For sandwiches and toast. Look for at least 3 grams of fibre per slice.

Fruits and Vegetables

- Berries - Blueberries, raspberries and blackberries are full of antioxidants.

- Cruciferous veggies - Broccoli, cauliflower, kale supply vitamin C, vitamin K, calcium.

- Tomatoes - Rich in lycopene, an antioxidant that may help protect skin from sun damage.

- Leafy greens - Spinach, kale, chard offer magnesium, iron, folate.

Herbs, Spices and Condiments

- Turmeric - Anti-inflammatory properties may help joint pain and heart health.

- Ginger - May aid nausea, digestion, inflammation. Add to tea, stir-fries.

- Garlic - Contains antimicrobial and immunity-boosting properties.

- Apple cider vinegar - Has uses for cooking, dressings, digestion and wellness tonics.

- Cinnamon - May help regulate blood sugar and has anti-inflammatory effects.

Beverages

- Green tea - Rich in antioxidants. Opt for decaf if caffeine sensitive.

- Herbal teas - Chamomile, peppermint can help soothe digestion.

- Bone broth - Sip warm as an anti-inflammatory tonic.

- Coconut water - Helps replenish fluids and electrolytes lost from hot flashes.

Other Essentials
- Nuts and seeds - Grab a handful for snacks, salads, oatmeal toppings.

- Canned fish - Salmon, tuna, sardines are ready protein sources.

- Nut butters - Look for brands with no added sugars. Spread on apples, toast.

- Hummus - For dipping veggies and crackers. Chickpeas provide protein, fibre.

- Frozen fruits and veggies - Have these on hand for smoothies, stir fries, soups.

Stocking your pantry and fridge with these nutritious staples can help provide the foundation for quick, healthy menopause-friendly meals and snacks.

Smart Grocery Shopping Tips for Menopausal Women

Grocery shopping during menopause requires some extra effort to ensure you are getting the right nutrients to support your changing body. Follow these comprehensive tips to shop smart during this transition.

Make a List and Stick To It

- Plan your meals and snacks for the week ahead of time
- Write down all ingredients needed to prepare those recipes to avoid buying extra items
- Check your pantry, fridge and freezer first to use up existing items before making your list
- Stick firmly to your list at the store to avoid impulse purchases

Shop the Perimeter First

- Spend most of your time shopping the outer aisles of the store
- This is where the healthiest whole food options are found - produce, lean proteins, low-fat dairy
- Limit time in inner aisles with processed and packaged foods
- Get in and out of these aisles efficiently

Load Up On Phytoestrogens

- Include foods like tofu, tempeh, flaxseeds, soybeans, oats, barley, legumes
- Phytoestrogens may help relieve menopausal symptoms like hot flashes
- Try edamame, miso soup, soy nuts, soy milk, lentil curry

Choose Healthy Fats

- Seek out omega-3 rich fats from fatty fish, avocados, nuts, seeds and oils

- Monounsaturated fats in olive oil, avocados and nuts help reduce inflammation
- Limit saturated fats found in red meat, butter, processed foods

Pick Calcium and Vitamin D Rich Foods

- Stock up on yoghourt, milk, cheese, leafy greens for bone health
- Get your vitamin D from eggs, salmon, tuna, fortified milk and safe sun
- Calcium and vitamin D together help prevent osteoporosis

Stay Hydrated

- Menopause hormones can cause bloating and fluid retention
- Counteract this by drinking plenty of water, herbal tea, coconut water
- Limit alcohol, sugary drinks and caffeine which can exacerbate dehydration

Read Labels for Hidden Sugars

- Avoid packaged snacks, cereals, drinks with added sugars
- Sugar crashes can worsen mood swings, insomnia and hot flashes
- Opt for low sugar snack options like nuts, seeds, cheese, Greek yoghourt

Shop With a Full Stomach

- Avoid shopping when hungry which leads to cravings and impulse buys
- Stick to your list after eating a meal or healthy snack beforehand

Follow these tips to optimise your grocery haul for a nutritious and balanced diet during menopause. Focus on perimeter whole foods, healthy fats, phytoestrogens and proper hydration to manage your symptoms gracefully.

Kitchen Tools to Simplify Your Cooking

Cooking nutritious meals consistently can be challenging during menopause. Having the right kitchen tools and appliances can streamline meal prep and reduce the burden of getting healthy food on the table. This guide explores tools to simplify cooking for menopausal women.

Food Processor

- Quickly chop, mince, shred, puree ingredients for sauces, dips, dressings
- Save time chopping veggies for soups, salads
- Grate cheese, shred cabbage for salads or slaws
- Puree beans into hummus

Immersion Blender

- Blend soups and sauces right in the pot

- Avoid transferring hot liquids to stand blender
- Puree vegetables into creamy soups without chunks
- Whip up dressings, dips, smoothies easily

Slow Cooker

- Prep ingredients in morning, come home to finished meal
- Tenderises lean meats like chicken breasts, flank steak
- Make big batches of chilli, soups, stews to freeze
- Avoid energy draining stove-top cooking

Air Fryer

- Circulates hot air to crisp up favourites like fries, nuggets
- Requires just a teaspoon of oil for crispy texture
- Cooks foods quickly with less fat than frying
- Make chicken wings, tofu, veggies

Stand Mixer

- Effortlessly knead dough for breads, pizza
- Whip up batters for muffins, cakes
- Mix and aerate ingredients thoroughly
- Attachments like whisk, paddle, dough hook

Food Steamer

- Gently cooks vegetables and fish en papillote
- Preserves nutrients compared to boiling
- Provides fast, healthy veggie side dishes
- Use rice cooker for grains too

Equipping your kitchen with handy appliances can remove some of the difficulty from preparing nutritious meals during menopause. Consider adding tools like food processors, immersion blenders, air fryers and more to simplify cooking.

Chapter 3

Breakfasts to Boost Your Day

Eating a nutritious breakfast is important for all women, but especially crucial during menopause. The right breakfast foods can help stabilise blood sugar, boost energy, improve mood, and provide key nutrients. Here are some great options:

Oatmeal

- Slow burning complex carbs provide steady energy
- Packed with soluble fibre to lower cholesterol
- Top with berries, nuts, seeds for extra nutrients
- Avoid instant oats with lots of added sugar

Eggs

- High in protein to keep you full and satisfied
- Contain vitamin D for bone health

- Choline promotes brain function and memory
- Make omelettes, frittatas loaded with veggies

Yogurt Parfaits
- Provides protein, calcium for bones, probiotics for gut
- Mix in berries, nuts, seeds, granola for crunch
- Skip premade parfaits high in added sugars

Tofu Scramble
- Plant-based protein from soy is rich in isoflavones
- Turmeric provides anti-inflammatory benefits
- Make a wrap with spinach and veggies for extra nutrients

Avocado Toast
- Healthy fats help absorb fat-soluble vitamins
- Fibre-rich whole grain or nut bread
- Top with smoked salmon, everything bagel seasoning

Smoothies

- Pack in fruits and veggies like spinach, kale
- Use yoghourt or milk for protein, calcium
- Nut butter provides staying power
- Avoid added sugars

Fuel your day right with a balanced breakfast containing protein, complex carbs and healthy fats. This provides steady energy, satisfies cravings and delivers key nutrients for menopausal women.

Energising Smoothie Bowls

Smoothie bowls are a nutritious and satisfying breakfast or snack for menopausal women seeking an energy boost. Blending fruits and veggies into a thick, creamy base and topping with crunchy, flavorful ingredients creates a delicious and customizable meal.

Base Ingredients

- Frozen banana - Provides creaminess and natural sweetness

- Frozen berries - Packed with antioxidants like raspberries, blueberries
- Leafy greens - Spinach, kale add nutrients without overpowering flavour
- Milk or yoghourt - Dairy provides protein, calcium for bone health
- Nut butter - Adds healthy fat for staying power
- Protein powder - Optionally add for extra protein

Toppings

- Fresh fruit - Strawberries, mango, pineapple for flavour and nutrients
- Nuts and seeds - Almonds, walnuts, chia, hemp hearts add crunch
- Coconut flakes - For texture and healthy fats
- Granola - Look for low-sugar varieties for crunch without added sugar
- Nut butter - Drizzle over for extra protein and healthy fat

Flavours

- Cocoa powder - For chocolate or mocha flavour
- Cinnamon - Warming spice to balance fruit flavours
- Vanilla extract - Add sweetness without sugar
- Ginger - Anti-inflammatory properties may ease joint pain
- Matcha - Provides antioxidant boost without caffeine jitters

Smoothie bowls allow you to customise both flavours and textures for a satisfying breakfast. Packed with protein, healthy fats, and fruits + veggies, they provide steady energy to power you through the day. Experiment with different ingredient combos to create your perfect energising blend.

Nutrient-Packed Overnight Oats

Overnight oats make for an easy, nutritious breakfast during menopause. Allowing oats to soak overnight softens them and enhances nutrient absorption. This lets you wake up to a ready-to-eat breakfast packed with fibre, protein and other key nutrients.

Base Ingredients

- Rolled or steel-cut oats - Choose unsweetened to avoid added sugar
- Milk - Dairy or non-dairy milk adds protein, calcium, vitamin D
- Greek yoghourt - Provides extra protein for staying power
- Chia seeds - A great source of omega-3s and fibre

Fruits and Veggies

- Berries - Antioxidant-rich blueberries, raspberries, strawberries
- Banana - Provides natural sweetness and potassium
- Apples - Chopped apples add fibre, vitamin C and flavour
- Spinach - Wilts into the oats and boosts nutrients

Nuts and Seeds

- Almonds - Packed with vitamin E, manganese and magnesium
- Walnuts - Supply omega-3s for brain, heart and skin health
- Flax or hemp seeds - Impart phytoestrogens, fibre, omega-3s
- Pumpkin seeds - Zinc helps support the immune system

Sweeteners

- Cinnamon - Adds warmth and balances blood sugar
- Maple syrup or honey - Use sparingly to lightly sweeten
- Vanilla extract - Provides flavour without added sugars
- Unsweetened coconut - Offers a subtle sweetness and crunch

Overnight oats offer an easy way to start the day with a balanced meal containing complex carbs, fibre, protein and healthy fats. Customise your oats by experimenting with different fruits, nuts, seeds and spices for a nutritious breakfast.

Protein-Packed Breakfasts to Fuel Your Morning

Getting adequate protein at breakfast is key for menopausal women. Protein provides steady energy, curbs cravings, maintains muscle mass and supports bone health as oestrogen levels decline. Here are some delicious high-protein breakfast options:

Greek Yoghourt
- Excellent source of protein, calcium, probiotics
- Opt for plain, unsweetened varieties
- Mix in fresh fruit, nuts, seeds, granola
- Makes a great base for parfaits too

Eggs

- One egg contains 6g high-quality protein
- Provide vitamin D and choline for brain function
- Prepare fried, scrambled, poached, in omelettes or frittatas
- Add veggies like spinach, tomatoes or avocado

Cottage Cheese
- Contains over 25g protein per cup
- Provides calcium for bone health
- Eat alone or use as base for bowls or parfaits
- Mix in fruits, nuts and seeds for added nutrition

Nut Butter Toast
- Look for nut butters with at least 5g protein per serving
- Contains healthy fats for hormone balance
- Spread on whole grain or seed bread
- Top with banana slices, cinnamon, raisins

Protein Smoothies

- Use protein powder or Greek yoghourt as a base
- Blend with milk, fruits, veggies, nut butter
- Keeps you full for hours compared to juice or fruit alone

Tofu Scramble
- Silken tofu contains about 10g protein per 1/2 cup
- Add turmeric, nutritional yeast, veggies for flavour
- Serve with avocado, sautéed greens, on toast

Fuel your mornings and prevent mid-day crashes by incorporating more protein at breakfast time. Combine high-protein foods like Greek yoghurt, eggs, cottage cheese or tofu with fruits, veggies and healthy fats.

Chapter 4

Vibrant Salads with Menopause-Friendly Ingredients

A vibrant salad with menopause-friendly ingredients can be a delicious and nutritious addition to a woman's diet during this significant life stage. Packed with essential nutrients, these salads can contribute to overall health, address specific menopausal symptoms, and offer a refreshing and satisfying meal. Here's a comprehensive guide on creating vibrant salads with menopause-friendly ingredients:

1. Base Greens:

Start with a nutrient-rich base of dark leafy greens like kale, spinach, arugula, or mixed salad greens. These greens are abundant in vitamins, minerals, and antioxidants, providing a solid foundation for a nutritious salad.

2. Lean Proteins:

Incorporate lean proteins to support muscle health and provide a feeling of fullness. Grilled chicken, salmon, tofu, chickpeas, or quinoa are excellent choices. These proteins also offer essential amino acids and omega-3 fatty acids, which are beneficial during menopause.

3. Calcium-Rich Additions:

Boost bone health by adding calcium-rich ingredients to your salad. Consider including dairy or plant-based alternatives like feta or goat cheese, almonds, chia seeds, or canned salmon with bones.

4. Colourful Vegetables:

Add a variety of colourful vegetables to your salad for a range of nutrients and antioxidants. Bell peppers, tomatoes, carrots, cucumbers, and beets are not only visually appealing but also provide essential vitamins and minerals.

5. Phytoestrogen-Rich Foods:

Incorporate foods rich in phytoestrogens, which may help balance hormonal fluctuations during menopause. Include ingredients like edamame, flaxseeds, sesame seeds, or tofu. These plant-based compounds can potentially offer relief from certain menopausal symptoms.

6. Healthy Fats:

Include sources of healthy fats for satiety and to support hormonal balance. Avocado, olive oil, nuts, and seeds are excellent choices. These fats contribute to heart health and can help manage weight, a common concern during menopause.

7. Whole Grains:

Incorporate whole grains for added fibre and sustained energy. Quinoa, farro, brown rice, or whole-grain couscous are nutritious options that complement the salad's texture and flavour while providing essential nutrients.

8. Herbs and Spices:

Enhance the flavour of your salad with fresh herbs and spices. Basil, cilantro, mint, and parsley not only add a burst of freshness but also offer anti-inflammatory properties. Consider spices like turmeric, which may help manage joint pain and inflammation.

9. Citrus Fruits:

Add a zing to your salad with citrus fruits like oranges, grapefruits, or mandarins. These fruits are rich in vitamin C, which supports the immune system and helps the body absorb iron from plant-based sources.

10. Dressing Options:

Opt for light and flavorful dressings made with olive oil, balsamic vinegar, lemon juice, or yoghurt. Homemade dressings allow for better control of ingredients and can be tailored to personal preferences. Avoiding excessive processed dressings can contribute to a healthier overall meal.

11. Hydrating Ingredients:

Include hydrating ingredients like cucumber or watermelon to enhance the salad's refreshing quality. Staying adequately hydrated is essential during menopause, and these ingredients contribute to overall fluid intake.

12. Mindful Portion Control:

Practise mindful portion control to avoid excessive calorie intake. While salads are nutrient-dense, being mindful of portion sizes helps maintain a balanced and healthy diet.

13. Customization for Individual Preferences:

Tailor your vibrant salad to individual preferences and dietary needs. Consider allergies, preferences, and cultural influences when selecting ingredients, ensuring a salad that is enjoyable and suited to personal tastes.

14. Consulting with Healthcare Professionals:

For women with specific dietary concerns or health conditions, consulting with healthcare professionals, such as registered dietitians or nutritionists, can provide personalised guidance and ensure the salad aligns with individual health goals.

In summary, creating vibrant salads with menopause-friendly ingredients involves a thoughtful selection of nutrient-dense components that address the unique nutritional needs of women during this life stage. These salads not only contribute to physical well-being but also provide a delicious and enjoyable way to support overall health and vitality during menopause.

Protein-Rich Lunch Bowl Ideas

Creating protein-rich lunch bowls for menopausal women is a great way to support their nutritional needs during this life stage. Here are some delicious and nutritious lunch bowl ideas:

1. Quinoa and Salmon Power Bowl:

- Base: Cooked quinoa.
- Protein: Grilled salmon or smoked salmon.
- Vegetables: Roasted Brussels sprouts, cherry tomatoes, and spinach.
- Extras: Avocado slices, pumpkin seeds, and a drizzle of lemon-tahini dressing.

2. Mediterranean Chickpea Salad Bowl:

- Base: Mixed greens or couscous.
- Protein: Chickpeas (roasted or marinated).
- Vegetables: Cucumber, red onion, cherry tomatoes, and Kalamata olives.
- Extras: Feta cheese, fresh herbs (like parsley or mint), and a Greek vinaigrette.

3. Chicken and Quinoa Veggie Bowl:

- Base: Tri-color quinoa.

- Protein: Grilled chicken breast.

- Vegetables: Roasted sweet potatoes, broccoli, and bell peppers.

- Extras: Feta cheese crumbles, sliced almonds, and a balsamic vinaigrette.

4. Tofu and Edamame Buddha Bowl:

- Base: Brown rice or mixed grains.

- Protein: Baked tofu cubes and steamed edamame.

- Vegetables: Shredded carrots, sliced radishes, and sautéed kale.

- Extras: Sesame seeds, avocado slices, and a soy-ginger dressing.

5. Shrimp and Avocado Quinoa Bowl:

- Base: Quinoa or cauliflower rice.

- Protein: Grilled shrimp.

- Vegetables: Sliced bell peppers, cherry tomatoes, and arugula.

- Extras: Sliced avocado, feta cheese, and a cilantro-lime dressing.

6. Salmon and Asparagus Grain Bowl:

- Base: Farro or wild rice.

- Protein: Baked or grilled salmon.

- Vegetables: Roasted asparagus, cherry tomatoes, and baby spinach.

- Extras: Sliced radishes, pine nuts, and a lemon-dill joghurt dressing.

Remember to customise these lunch bowl ideas based on individual preferences and dietary restrictions. These protein-rich bowls offer a balance of nutrients, including essential proteins, fibre, and healthy fats, making them ideal for supporting the nutritional needs of menopausal women.

Quick and Healthy Soup Recipes

1. Quinoa and Chickpea Power Bowl:

- Procedure: Cook quinoa and mix with roasted chickpeas, cherry tomatoes, cucumber, and feta cheese. Drizzle with olive oil and lemon juice.

2. Salmon and Avocado Quinoa Bowl:

- Procedure: Grill salmon and serve over a bed of cooked quinoa. Top with avocado slices, arugula, and a lemon-tahini dressing.

3. Lentil and Vegetable Buddha Bowl:

- Procedure: Cook lentils and arrange in a bowl with roasted sweet potatoes, broccoli, and kale. Add a dollop of Greek yoghurt and a sprinkle of pumpkin seeds.

4. Turkey and Quinoa Stuffed Peppers:

- Procedure: Mix cooked quinoa with ground turkey, black beans, corn, and salsa. Stuff bell peppers and bake until tender.

5. Tofu and Edamame Noodle Bowl:

- Procedure: Stir-fry tofu and edamame with colourful vegetables. Toss with cooked soba noodles and a ginger-soy sauce.

6. Chicken and Spinach Salad Bowl:

- Procedure: Grill chicken and slice. Arrange over a bed of fresh spinach with cherry tomatoes, sliced almonds, and a balsamic vinaigrette.

7. Greek Chickpea Salad Bowl:

- Procedure: Combine chickpeas with cucumber, cherry tomatoes, red onion, olives, and feta cheese. Toss in olive oil and lemon juice.

8. Shrimp and Quinoa Stir-Fry Bowl:

- Procedure: Stir-fry shrimp with colourful vegetables and mix with cooked quinoa. Season with soy sauce and a hint of sesame oil.

9. Egg and Avocado Breakfast Bowl:

- Procedure: Poach eggs and serve over a quinoa and black bean base. Top with sliced avocado, salsa, and a sprinkle of feta cheese.

10. Spinach and Walnut Pesto Pasta Bowl:

- Procedure: Blend spinach and walnut pesto. Toss with whole-grain pasta, cherry tomatoes, and grilled chicken or tofu.

Adjust portions according to individual preferences and dietary needs. These lunch bowl ideas provide a balance of protein, fibre, and essential nutrients, contributing to overall well-being during menopause.

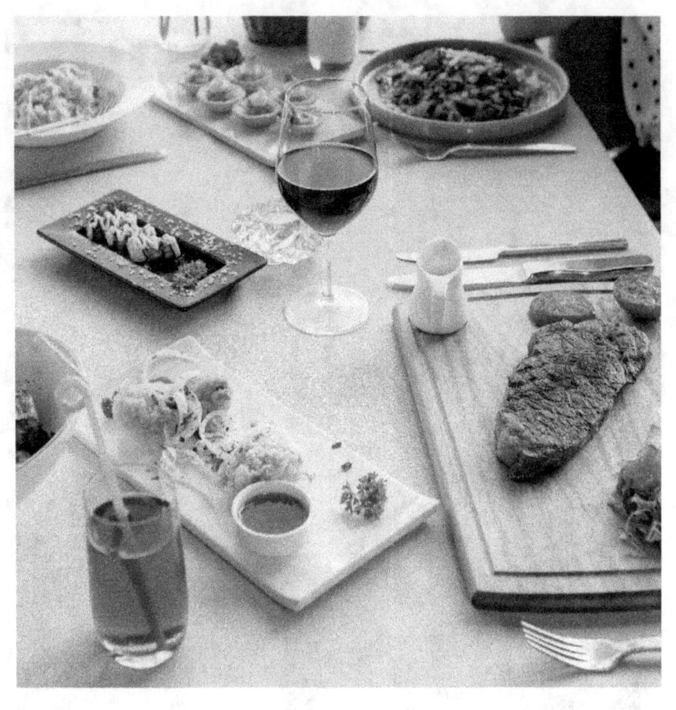

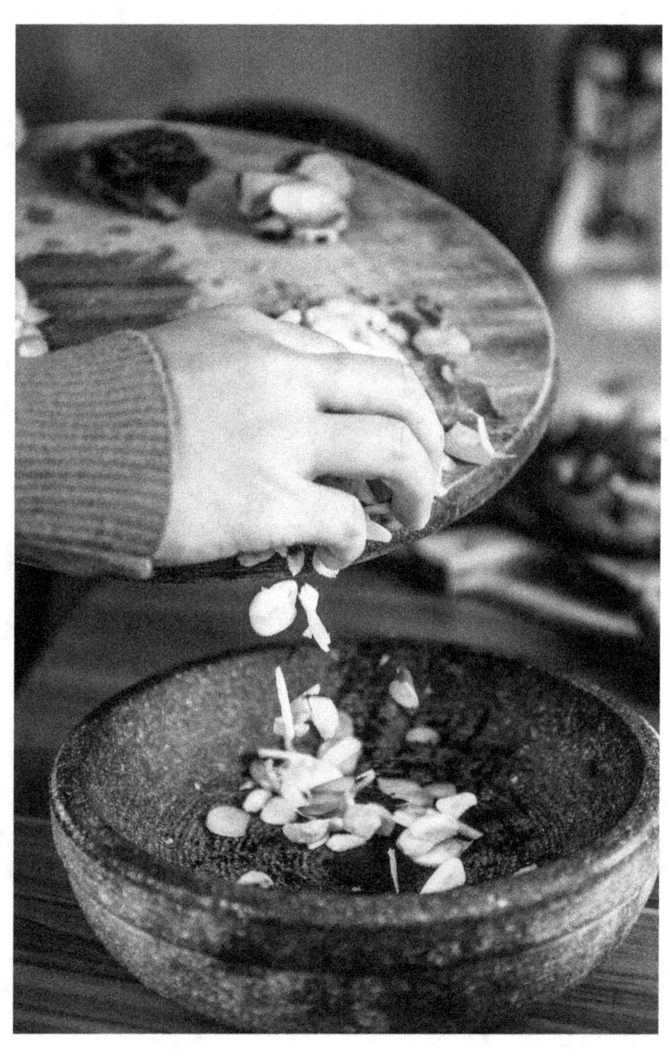

Chapter 5

Satisfying Snacks to Tame Menopausal Cravings

Taming menopausal cravings requires satisfying snacks that provide a combination of nutrients to support overall health. Here are some snack ideas tailored to help curb cravings during menopause:

1. Greek Yogurt Parfait:

- Layer Greek yoghurt with fresh berries, granola, and a drizzle of honey. This snack is rich in protein, probiotics, and antioxidants.

2. Hummus and Veggie Sticks:

- Dip carrot, cucumber, and bell pepper sticks in hummus. Hummus provides protein and healthy fats, while veggies offer vitamins and fibre.

3. Nuts and Dried Fruits Mix:

   - Combine a mix of almonds, walnuts, and dried fruits like apricots or cranberries. This snack provides a satisfying crunch and a balance of protein and natural sugars.

4. Cottage Cheese with Pineapple:

   - Enjoy a bowl of cottage cheese with fresh pineapple chunks. Cottage cheese is a good source of protein, and pineapple adds natural sweetness.

5. Dark Chocolate and Almond Clusters:

   - Create clusters by combining dark chocolate with almonds. Dark chocolate satisfies sweet cravings, and almonds provide a dose of healthy fats and protein.

6. Whole Grain Crackers with Cheese:

   - Pair whole grain crackers with cheese slices. This snack offers a combination of fibre, protein, and calcium.

7. Roasted Chickpeas:

   - Roast chickpeas with a mix of spices for a crunchy and satisfying snack. Chickpeas provide protein and fibre, helping to keep you full.

8. Smoothie Bowl:

   - Blend a smoothie with fruits, yoghurt, and a handful of greens. Top with granola and chia seeds for added texture and nutrients.

9. Avocado Toast:

   - Spread mashed avocado on whole grain toast and sprinkle with sea salt. Avocados are rich in healthy fats and fibre.

10. Edamame Pods:

   - Steam edamame pods and lightly salt them. Edamame is a good source of plant-based protein and fibre.

11. Apple Slices with Nut Butter:

- Slice apples and dip them in almond or peanut butter. The combination of sweet and savoury satisfies cravings while providing a mix of nutrients.

12. Trail Mix with Seeds:

- Create a trail mix with a variety of nuts, seeds, and a touch of dark chocolate. Seeds add an extra boost of nutrients and texture.

Remember to stay hydrated and choose snacks that provide a balance of protein, healthy fats, and carbohydrates to keep energy levels stable and cravings in check during the menopausal journey.

Healthy Trail Mix and Snack Bars

Creating healthy trail mix and snack bars for menopausal women involves selecting nutrient-dense ingredients that support overall health and address specific nutritional needs during this life stage. Here are ideas for both:

Healthy Trail Mix:

1. Nuts Mix:

- Almonds, walnuts, and pistachios provide healthy fats, omega-3s, and protein.

2. Dried Fruits:

- Apricots, cranberries, and raisins offer natural sweetness and antioxidants.

3. Seeds:

- Pumpkin seeds and sunflower seeds contribute additional healthy fats and nutrients.

4. Dark Chocolate:

- Opt for dark chocolate chips for a satisfying sweet touch and antioxidants.

5. Coconut Flakes:

- Unsweetened coconut adds flavour and texture without excess sugar.

Snack Bar Ideas:

1. Nutty Energy Bars:

- Blend almonds, cashews, and dates in a food processor. Add chia seeds, dried fruits, and a touch of honey. Press into bars and refrigerate.

2. Quinoa Crunch Bars:

- Mix popped quinoa, nuts, seeds, and dried fruits. Bind with a mixture of almond butter and honey. Press into bars and let them set.

3. Protein-Packed Peanut Butter Bars:

- Combine rolled oats, peanut butter, protein powder, and a drizzle of maple syrup. Press into bars and refrigerate.

4. Chia Seed Bliss Bars:

- Mix chia seeds, almond butter, honey, and a pinch of cinnamon. Allow the mixture to set in the refrigerator before cutting into bars.

5. Fruit and Nut Bars:

- Blend dates, dried fruits, almonds, and a hint of vanilla. Press into bars and refrigerate until firm.

6. No-Bake Almond Joy Bars:

- Combine shredded coconut, almonds, dates, and a layer of dark chocolate. Chill until set and cut into bars.

7. Pumpkin Spice Energy Bars:

- Mix rolled oats, pumpkin puree, nuts, and a blend of spices. Press into bars and refrigerate.

8. Cranberry Almond Protein Bars:

- Blend almonds, dried cranberries, protein powder, and a touch of honey. Shape into bars and chill.

Tips:

- Portion Control: While these snacks are healthy, portion control is key. Pre-portion your trail mix and bars to avoid overeating.

-Hydration: Stay well-hydrated. Consider including water-rich ingredients like coconut and hydrating fruits.

-Whole Ingredients: Choose whole, minimally processed ingredients for optimal nutrition.

Customise these recipes based on taste preferences, dietary restrictions, and nutritional needs. These trail mix and snack bars offer a convenient and nourishing option for menopausal women seeking a healthy and satisfying snack.

Homemade Energy Bites and Sweets

Creating homemade energy bites and sweets for menopausal women involves selecting ingredients that provide sustained energy, address nutritional needs, and offer a delightful treat. Here are some recipes to try:

Homemade Energy Bites:

1. Cocoa Almond Bliss Bites:

- Blend almonds, dates, cocoa powder, and a touch of vanilla. Roll into bite-sized balls and refrigerate.

2. Chia Seed and Berry Bites:

- Mix chia seeds, dried berries, almond butter, and a drizzle of honey. Form into small bites and chill.

3. Peanut Butter Banana Energy Bites:

- Combine mashed bananas, oats, peanut butter, and a sprinkle of cinnamon. Shape into bites and refrigerate.

4. Coconut Matcha Energy Bites:

- Blend shredded coconut, almonds, matcha powder, and dates. Roll into bites and refrigerate.

5. Apricot and Walnut Energy Bites:

- Process dried apricots, walnuts, and a hint of orange zest. Shape into bite-sized balls and chill.

Homemade Sweets:

1. Dark Chocolate-Dipped Strawberries:

- Dip fresh strawberries in melted dark chocolate. Allow them to sit in the refrigerator.

2. Yoghourt-Covered Blueberries:

- Dip blueberries in Greek yoghurt and freeze until solid for a refreshing sweet treat.

3. Frozen Banana Pops:

- Skewer banana slices and dip in melted dark chocolate. Freeze for a cool and satisfying snack.

4. Almond Butter-Stuffed Dates:

- Remove the pits from dates and stuff with almond butter. Sprinkle with chopped nuts or coconut.

5. Cinnamon Baked Apples:

- Slice apples and toss with cinnamon. Bake until tender for a warm and comforting sweet.

Tips:

-Balanced Ingredients: Include a mix of healthy fats, proteins, and carbohydrates for sustained energy.

-Hydrating Elements: Incorporate fruits with high water content for hydration, like berries and watermelon.

-Portion Control: Despite their healthfulness, be mindful of portion sizes to manage calorie intake.

-Experiment with Flavors: Add spices like cinnamon, nutmeg, or a hint of sea salt for flavour variety.

These homemade energy bites and sweets offer a combination of nutritional benefits and indulgence, making them ideal for menopausal women seeking a delightful and nourishing treat.

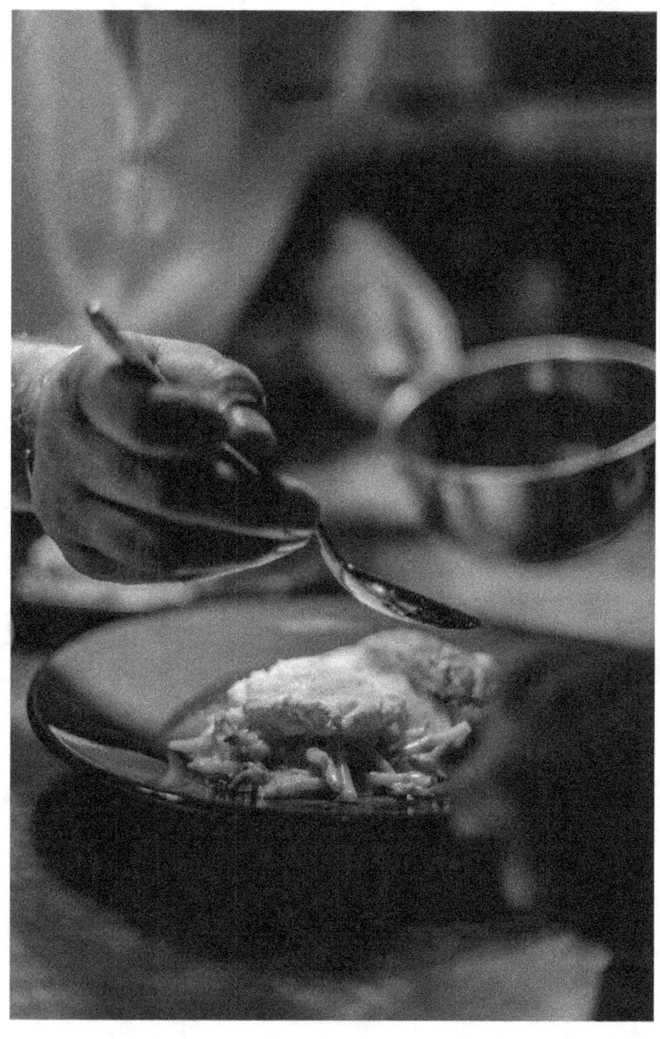

Chapter 6

Dinner Delights for Balanced Nutrition

Creating dinner delights for balanced nutrition during menopause involves incorporating a mix of nutrients to support overall health. Here are some ideas for well-rounded and delicious dinners:

Grilled Salmon with Quinoa and Roasted Vegetables:

- Grill salmon seasoned with herbs and lemon. Serve it over a bed of cooked quinoa and roasted vegetables like broccoli, bell peppers, and sweet potatoes. This dish provides omega-3 fatty acids, protein, and a variety of vitamins and minerals.

Chickpea and Vegetable Stir-Fry:

- Stir-fry chickpeas with a colourful mix of vegetables like kale, bell peppers, and snap peas. Season with ginger, garlic, and low-sodium soy sauce. Serve over brown rice or cauliflower rice for a plant-based, protein-rich meal.

Mediterranean Chicken Bowl:

- Marinate chicken in olive oil, lemon, and Mediterranean spices before grilling. Serve over a base of whole grains like farro or quinoa, and top with a Greek salad of cucumbers, tomatoes, olives, and feta. This meal offers a balance of lean protein, whole grains, and healthy fats.

Lentil and Vegetable Curry:

- Make a hearty lentil and vegetable curry with tomatoes, spinach, and spices. Serve over brown rice or quinoa for a plant-based dinner rich in protein, fibre, and essential nutrients.

Baked Cod with Roasted Brussels Sprouts and Sweet Potatoes:

- Season cod fillets with herbs and bake. Roast Brussels sprouts and sweet potatoes as sides. This dinner is high in omega-3s, fibre, and vitamins.

Quinoa-Stuffed Bell Peppers:

- Mix cooked quinoa with black beans, corn, tomatoes, and spices. Stuff bell peppers and bake until tender. This vegetarian dish provides a complete protein source and a variety of nutrients.

Turkey and Vegetable Skewers:

- Thread turkey chunks, cherry tomatoes, zucchini, and mushrooms onto skewers. Grill or bake, and serve over a bulgur or couscous salad. This meal offers lean protein, fibre, and a mix of vegetables.

Cauliflower and Chickpea Curry:

- Make a curry with cauliflower, chickpeas, and spinach. Serve over brown rice or cauliflower rice for a low-carb option. This dish is rich in plant-based protein, fibre, and antioxidants.

Quinoa and Broccoli Casserole:

- Combine cooked quinoa with steamed broccoli, chicken breast, and a light cheese sauce. Bake until bubbly for a comforting and balanced meal.

Shrimp and Avocado Salad:

- Toss grilled shrimp with mixed greens, avocado, cherry tomatoes, and a citrus vinaigrette. This salad provides a dose of healthy fats, protein, and a variety of vitamins.

Tips:

-Colourful Plate: Aim for a colourful plate with a variety of vegetables to ensure a range of nutrients.

-Portion Control: Be mindful of portion sizes to maintain a healthy balance of nutrients without overeating.

-Hydration: Accompany your meal with water or herbal tea to stay hydrated.

By incorporating a variety of nutrient-dense ingredients, these dinner ideas cater to the specific nutritional needs of menopausal women, promoting overall well-being.

Lean Protein Recipes for Dinner

Incorporating lean protein into dinner is crucial for menopausal women to support muscle health and overall well-being. Here are some delicious and nutritious lean protein recipes:

Grilled Chicken Salad with Quinoa:
- Marinate chicken breasts in olive oil, lemon juice, and herbs. Grill until cooked through and

slice. Serve over a bed of mixed greens, quinoa, cherry tomatoes, cucumbers, and a light vinaigrette.

Baked Salmon with Asparagus and Lemon:

- Season salmon fillets with herbs and a squeeze of lemon. Bake alongside fresh asparagus. This dish is rich in omega-3 fatty acids and provides a light and flavorful dinner.

Turkey and Vegetable Stir-Fry:

- Stir-fry lean ground turkey with an array of colourful vegetables like bell peppers, broccoli, and snap peas. Season with garlic, ginger, and low-sodium soy sauce. Serve over brown rice or cauliflower rice.

Greek Yogurt and Herb-Marinated Grilled Chicken:

- Marinate chicken in a mixture of Greek yoghurt, garlic, lemon, and herbs. Grill until cooked through. Serve with a side of roasted sweet potatoes and steamed green beans.

Quinoa and Black Bean Stuffed Peppers:
- Mix cooked quinoa with black beans, corn, tomatoes, and spices. Stuff bell peppers and bake until tender. Top with a dollop of Greek yoghurt and fresh cilantro.

Grilled Shrimp Skewers with Mango Salsa:
- Thread shrimp on skewers and grill until opaque. Serve with a refreshing mango salsa made with diced mango, red onion, cilantro, and lime juice.

Lemon Herb Baked Cod:
- Season cod fillets with a mix of lemon, garlic, and herbs. Bake until the fish flakes easily. Pair with a side of steamed broccoli and quinoa for a light and nutritious dinner.

Chicken and Vegetable Kabobs:

- Thread chicken breast chunks, cherry tomatoes, zucchini, and mushrooms onto skewers. Grill until the chicken is cooked through. Serve with a side of quinoa or a green salad.

Tofu and Vegetable Stir-Fry:
- Cube tofu and stir-fry with a colourful mix of vegetables like bell peppers, broccoli, and carrots. Season with a light soy or teriyaki sauce. Serve over brown rice or cauliflower rice.

Greek Salad with Grilled Chicken:
- Grill chicken breasts seasoned with oregano and lemon. Slice and serve over a Greek salad with tomatoes, cucumbers, olives, and feta cheese. Drizzle with olive oil and balsamic vinegar.

Tips:
- Lean Cuts: Opt for lean cuts of meat and skinless poultry to reduce saturated fat intake.

-Plant-Based Proteins: Incorporate plant-based proteins like tofu, black beans, and quinoa for variety.

-Balanced Meals: Combine lean proteins with a variety of colourful vegetables and whole grains for a balanced meal.

These lean protein recipes provide a mix of flavours and nutrients, supporting menopausal women in maintaining muscle health and meeting their dietary needs.

Wholesome Grain and Vegetable Combinations

Welcoming wholesome grains and vegetables into meals is essential for menopausal women to support overall health, provide essential nutrients, and manage weight. Here are some delicious grain and vegetable combinations:

Quinoa and Roasted Vegetable Bowl:

- Roast a mix of colourful vegetables such as sweet potatoes, bell peppers, and zucchini. Serve over a bed of cooked quinoa. Drizzle with olive oil and sprinkle with fresh herbs.

Brown Rice Stir-Fry with Tofu and Broccoli:

- Stir-fry tofu cubes with broccoli florets, snap peas, and carrots. Toss with cooked brown rice and a savoury soy or teriyaki sauce.

Farro Salad with Mediterranean Vegetables:

- Cook farro and mix with cherry tomatoes, cucumbers, olives, and feta cheese. Dress with a lemon vinaigrette for a refreshing Mediterranean-inspired dish.

Lentil and Vegetable Curry with Brown Rice:

- Prepare a hearty lentil and vegetable curry with tomatoes, spinach, and spices. Serve over brown rice for a protein-packed, fibre-rich meal.

Quinoa and Black Bean Stuffed Bell Peppers:

- Mix cooked quinoa with black beans, corn, tomatoes, and spices. Stuff bell peppers and bake until tender. Top with a dollop of Greek yoghurt and fresh cilantro.

Whole Wheat Pasta Primavera:

- Toss whole wheat pasta with a medley of sautéed vegetables like cherry tomatoes, bell peppers, and asparagus. Drizzle with olive oil and sprinkle with Parmesan cheese.

Barley and Roasted Vegetable Salad:

- Roast a variety of vegetables like eggplant, cherry tomatoes, and red onions. Mix with cooked barley and a balsamic vinaigrette for a satisfying and nutritious salad.

Cauliflower Fried Rice:

- Pulse cauliflower in a food processor to create rice-sized pieces. Stir-fry with colourful vegetables, scrambled eggs, and soy sauce for a low-carb alternative to traditional fried rice.

Bulgur and Chickpea Pilaf with Spinach:
- Cook bulgur and mix with chickpeas, sautéed spinach, and a squeeze of lemon. This combination offers a good balance of protein, fibre, and vitamins.

Spaghetti Squash with Tomato and Basil Sauce:
- Roast spaghetti squash and top with a homemade tomato and basil sauce. This low-carb alternative to pasta is rich in vitamins and antioxidants.

Tips:
-Varied Vegetables: Include a variety of colourful vegetables to ensure a diverse range of nutrients.

-Whole Grains: Choose whole grains like quinoa, brown rice, farro, or barley for added fibre and nutritional benefits.

-Herbs and Spices: Enhance flavours with herbs and spices instead of excessive salt or creamy sauces.

These wholesome grain and vegetable combinations offer a range of nutrients crucial for menopausal women, supporting their health and well-being during this transformative phase of life.

One-Pot Wonders for Easy Cleanup

Quinoa Primavera:
Sauté colourful bell peppers, cherry tomatoes, and zucchini in a pot. Add quinoa, vegetable broth, and your favourite herbs. Simmer until quinoa is cooked. Top with fresh basil and a

sprinkle of Parmesan for a quick and nutritious one-pot meal.

Chicken and Vegetable Curry:

Cook diced chicken, cauliflower, and spinach in a pot with curry spices and coconut milk. Simmer until the flavours meld. Serve over brown rice for a flavorful and comforting dinner with minimal cleanup.

Lemon Garlic Shrimp Pasta:

Cook whole wheat spaghetti with shrimp, cherry tomatoes, and spinach in a pot. Add a zesty sauce of garlic, lemon, and olive oil. Toss everything in one pot for a quick, light, and satisfying meal.

Mushroom and Spinach Risotto:

Sauté mushrooms and spinach in a pot, add Arborio rice, and gradually stir in vegetable broth. Let it simmer until the rice is creamy. Garnish with Parmesan for a comforting risotto without the fuss.

One-Pan Baked Salmon with Vegetables:

Place salmon fillets on a sheet pan surrounded by a mix of chopped broccoli, carrots, and potatoes. Drizzle with olive oil, season, and bake for an easy, well-balanced dinner with minimal cleanup.

Tofu and Vegetable Stir-Fry:

Stir-fry tofu with an assortment of colourful vegetables in a wok or deep skillet. Add soy sauce, ginger, and garlic for flavour. Serve over brown rice or quinoa for a quick and healthy one-pan dish.

Spicy Sausage and Orzo Skillet:

Brown spicy sausage in a skillet, add orzo, diced tomatoes, and a mix of bell peppers. Simmer until the orzo is cooked, and you have a flavorful one-pot meal that's both satisfying and easy to clean up.

Cajun Chickpea and Rice Skillet:

Sauté Cajun-spiced chickpeas with bell peppers and onions in a skillet. Add cooked rice and a splash of vegetable broth. Simmer until heated through for a spicy and convenient one-pot dinner.

Vegetable and Lentil Soup:
Combine lentils, a variety of chopped vegetables, and vegetable broth in a pot. Simmer until the lentils are tender. This hearty soup is not only nutritious but also offers easy cleanup.

Pesto Zucchini Noodles with Cherry Tomatoes:
Sauté zucchini noodles with cherry tomatoes in a skillet. Add a dollop of pesto and toss until everything is coated. A light and fresh dish that's both easy to prepare and clean up.

Chapter 7

Meal Planning and Prep Tips for Busy Menopausal Women

Streamlined Grocery Shopping:

Plan meals ahead and create a detailed shopping list. Organise it by sections in the store to save time. Consider online grocery shopping or delivery services for added convenience.

Batch Cooking:

Prepare large batches of staple items like grains, proteins, and sauces on the weekends. This allows for easy assembly during busy weekdays, cutting down daily cooking time.

Freezer-Friendly Meals:

Prepare freezer-friendly meals in advance. Soups, casseroles, and marinated proteins can be portioned and stored for quick and easy meals when time is limited.

Pre-Cut and Washed Vegetables:

Purchase pre-cut and washed vegetables or take some time during the week to prep them. Having veggies ready to go makes it easier to incorporate them into meals.

Simple One-Pot Meals:

Opt for one-pot or sheet pan meals that minimise cleanup. This not only saves time but also reduces the number of dishes to wash.

Flexible Meal Plans:

Create a flexible meal plan for the week. Include simple recipes that share ingredients to minimise waste and make cooking more efficient.

Healthy Snack Prep:

Prep healthy snacks like cut fruits, vegetables, and portioned nuts in advance. Having nutritious snacks readily available helps curb cravings and maintains energy levels.

Use Convenience Items Wisely:

Incorporate healthy convenience items like pre-cooked grains, canned beans, and pre-washed greens. These can significantly cut down on cooking time.

Multitasking Cooking:

Utilise downtime in the kitchen efficiently. While one item is cooking, work on prepping the next. This multitasking approach streamlines the overall cooking process.

Slow Cooker and Instant Pot Recipes:

Explore slow cooker or Instant Pot recipes. These appliances allow for hands-free cooking and often result in flavorful, tender dishes with minimal effort.

Portion Control and Storage:

Portion meals as you prepare them and store them in individual containers. This makes it easy to grab a pre-portioned, balanced meal when needed.

Delegate and Share Responsibilities:
Involve family members in meal planning and preparation. Delegate tasks or consider sharing cooking responsibilities to lighten the load.

Self-Care and Mindful Eating:
Prioritise self-care, including mindful eating. Take the time to enjoy meals without distractions, promoting better digestion and overall well-being.

Adapt and Simplify:
Be flexible with meal plans. If a day becomes busier than expected, have a repertoire of quick and simple recipes as backups.

Stay Hydrated:

Remember to stay hydrated. Prepare infused water or herbal teas in advance for a refreshing and healthful beverage option.

By implementing these meal planning and prep tips, busy menopausal women can maintain a nutritious and balanced diet while efficiently managing their time and energy.

Weekly Meal Planning Strategies

Theme Nights:
Assign specific themes to each day of the week. For example, have Meatless Monday, Taco Tuesday, or Stir-Fry Friday. This adds variety and simplifies decision-making.

Batch Cooking on Weekends:
Devote some time on weekends to batch cooking. Prepare staple items like grilled chicken, quinoa, and roasted vegetables that can be used in different combinations throughout the week.

Seasonal and Local Ingredients:

Plan meals around seasonal and local ingredients. This ensures freshness, supports local businesses, and introduces a variety of nutrients into the diet.

Create a Flexible Menu:

Develop a menu for the week but keep it flexible. This allows for adjustments based on unexpected events or changing preferences.

Balance Macronutrients

Ensure a balance of macronutrients (proteins, fats, and carbohydrates) in each meal. This helps maintain energy levels and provides essential nutrients.

Mindful Portioning:

Mindfully portion meals to avoid overeating. Use smaller plates to encourage proper portion sizes and reduce food waste.

Plan for Leftovers:

Incorporate meals that are conducive to leftovers. This reduces the need for daily cooking and ensures there's always a ready-made option.

Quick and Easy Recipes:

Include quick and easy recipes in your plan for busier days. This could be a simple stir-fry, a grain bowl, or a salad with pre-prepped ingredients.

Utilise Frozen Ingredients:

Keep a stock of frozen fruits, vegetables, and proteins. These items are convenient and have a longer shelf life, providing flexibility in meal planning.

Family Involvement:

Involve family members in meal planning. Take preferences into account and share the responsibility of preparing meals.

Plan for Snacks:

Include snacks in your meal plan. Have a mix of healthy options like cut vegetables, nuts, or yoghourt to satisfy cravings between meals.

Prep-Ahead Breakfasts:

Prepare breakfast items in advance. Overnight oats, chia seed puddings, or pre-made smoothie packs can be excellent time-savers.

Rotation of Favourites:

Rotate favourite meals within the week. This ensures a balance between variety and familiarity, making mealtime enjoyable.

Check Pantry and Fridge:

Before planning, take stock of what's in your pantry and fridge. This helps reduce food waste and ensures you use existing ingredients.

Hydration Planning:

Include hydration in your plan. Have water, herbal teas, or infused water readily available throughout the day.

Consider Dietary Preferences and Restrictions:
Factor in any dietary preferences or restrictions when planning meals. This ensures that everyone's needs are met.

Adapting these weekly meal planning strategies can help menopausal women maintain a nutritious and well-rounded diet while efficiently managing their time and resources.

Batch Cooking and Freezing for Convenience

Batch Cooking Essentials:
Designate a day for batch cooking. Prepare large quantities of staple items like grilled chicken, brown rice, quinoa, and roasted

vegetables. These can serve as the base for various meals throughout the week.

Freeze in Portions:

Divide batch-cooked items into individual or family-sized portions before freezing. This facilitates easy thawing and minimises food wastage.

Sauces and Marinades:

Prepare versatile sauces and marinades in batches. Freeze them in ice cube trays for easy portioning. These can be quickly added to meals for enhanced flavour.

Soup and Stew Freezing:

Prepare hearty soups and stews in large batches. Portion them into freezer-safe containers for convenient, ready-to-heat meals.

Marinated Proteins:

Marinate proteins like chicken, fish, or tofu in bulk. Freeze them in separate bags with the marinade. Thaw and cook for a quick and flavorful meal.

Casserole Dishes:

Make casseroles and one-dish meals in large quantities. Portion and freeze them for easy reheating when time is limited.

Pre-Portioned Smoothie Packs:

Prepare and freeze smoothie ingredients in individual packs. This includes fruits, greens, and any additional add-ins. In the morning, blend with liquid for a quick and nutritious breakfast.

Labelling and Dating:

Label each container with the name of the dish and the date it was prepared. This ensures you use items before they lose quality.

Freezer-Friendly Snacks:

Make snacks like energy bites, muffins, or granola bars in bulk. Freeze them individually for grab-and-go convenience.

Fruit and Vegetable Preservation:
Freeze excess fruits and vegetables. Berries, sliced bananas, and chopped veggies can be used in smoothies or added to recipes directly from the freezer.

Pre-Portioned Grains:
Cook and freeze grains like brown rice, quinoa, or couscous in portioned bags. These can be quickly reheated for a side dish or added to salads and bowls.

Thawing Strategies:
Plan ahead for thawing. Transfer frozen items to the refrigerator the night before or use the defrost setting on your microwave for quicker thawing.

Inventory Management:

Keep an inventory of items in your freezer. Regularly update it to avoid overcrowding and to use older items first.

Rotating Stock:

Practise a "first in, first out" approach. This ensures that older frozen items are used before newer ones, maintaining optimal freshness.

Customizable Frozen Meal Kits:

Create frozen meal kits by combining pre-cooked proteins, grains, and vegetables. Label them for easy identification and mix-and-match flexibility.

Easy-to-Reheat Containers:

Invest in microwave-safe and oven-safe containers for easy reheating. This eliminates the need for transferring food to different dishes.

Batch cooking and freezing are invaluable strategies for menopausal women, providing the convenience of ready-made meals while allowing for better control over ingredients and nutritional content.

Creating a Sustainable Meal Routine

Mindful Planning:

Take a mindful approach to meal planning. Consider dietary preferences, nutritional needs, and sustainable food choices. Plan meals that align with personal values and health goals.

Seasonal Eating:

Base meals on seasonal and locally available produce. This not only supports local farmers but also ensures a variety of fresh, nutrient-dense foods.

Plant-Centric Emphasis:

Place a strong emphasis on plant-based meals. Incorporate a variety of vegetables, legumes, whole grains, and nuts to enhance nutritional intake and support overall well-being.

Mindful Eating Practices:

Practise mindful eating. Slow down, savour each bite, and listen to hunger and fullness cues. This fosters a healthier relationship with food and encourages better digestion.

Flexibility in Meal Plans:

Create flexible meal plans that can adapt to changing schedules. Allow room for improvisation, accommodating busy days without compromising nutrition.

Reducing Food Waste:

Minimise food waste by planning meals that use ingredients efficiently. Incorporate leftovers into subsequent meals, and freeze excess portions for future use.

Sustainable Proteins:

Choose sustainable protein sources such as plant-based proteins, responsibly sourced fish, and ethically raised poultry. This reduces the environmental impact of the diet.

Mindful Meat Consumption:

If consuming meat, do so mindfully. Opt for lean cuts and smaller portions, emphasising quality over quantity. Consider meatless days to further reduce environmental impact.

Local and Ethical Sourcing:

Prioritise local and ethically sourced ingredients. Support farmers' markets and local suppliers to reduce the carbon footprint of your meals.

Meal Diversity:

Ensure a diverse range of foods in your meals. This not only contributes to a well-balanced diet but also promotes gut health and overall vitality.

Homemade Convenience Foods:

Make your own convenience foods to reduce reliance on processed, packaged items. This includes sauces, dressings, and snacks prepared with whole, minimally processed ingredients.

Mindful Hydration:

Stay hydrated with mindful beverage choices. Choose water, herbal teas, and infused waters over sugary drinks to support overall health.

Culinary Exploration:

Embrace culinary exploration by trying new recipes and cooking techniques. This adds variety to the diet and makes mealtime more enjoyable.

Family Involvement:

Involve family members in meal planning and preparation. Share responsibilities and gather input to create a shared commitment to sustainable and healthy eating.

Reflect and Adjust:

Regularly reflect on your meal routine. Assess what works well and what can be improved. Make adjustments as needed to create a sustainable and enjoyable approach to eating.

By incorporating these practices, menopausal women can create a sustainable meal routine that aligns with their health goals, supports the environment, and fosters a positive relationship with food.

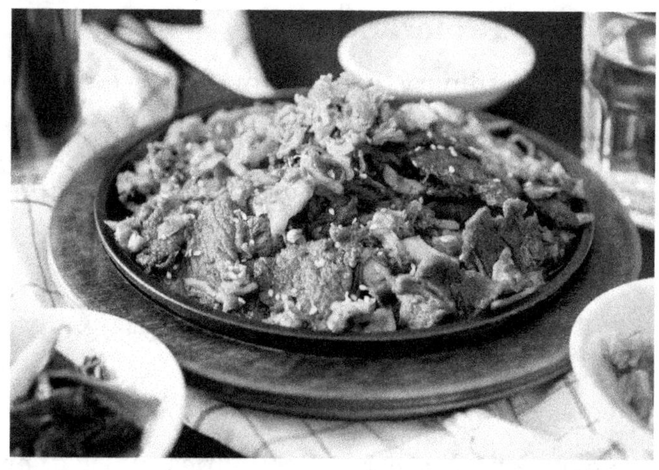

Chapter 8

Tracking Your Menopause Manifesto Diet Journey

Making dietary changes to manage menopausal symptoms and optimise wellbeing is extremely worthwhile, but also challenging. Tracking your progress provides accountability, identifies effective approaches, and celebrates small wins - helping to motivate you through this transition. This guide explores comprehensive strategies to track your Menopause Manifesto diet over the long-term.

Set Specific Goals

Be very clear on why you are changing your diet and set related S.M.A.R.T. goals that are Specific, Measurable, Achievable, Relevant and Time-bound. Do you hope to reduce hot flashes, stabilise energy, improve mood, manage weight, or boost nutrition? Outline explicit goals like "Eat 25-30g protein, 10g fibre, and 3 servings fruits/veggies at each meal daily for reduced cravings and crashes."

Weigh and Measure Portions

Getting familiar with proper portion sizes for whole foods versus processed items takes guesswork out of building balanced meals and snacks. Invest in a food scale and measure cups to quantify ounces of proteins, cups of grains and dairy, teaspoon oils. Compare the volume metrics to common household items like a tennis ball or deck of cards.

Log Food Intake

Recording all food and drinks consumed each day provides concrete data to analyse. Capture meals, snacks, ingredients, brands, cooking methods, and portion sizes. Free apps like MyFitnessPal or Cronometer make tracking easy with extensive databases. Also log timing, hunger/fullness levels before/after eating, exercise duration, mood and symptom severity.

Take Before Photos

Photos provide visible proof of changes over time that scales don't show - like muscle tone, bloating and skin/hair quality. Take front, side and back photos in tight clothing like sports bras and shorts. Use consistent lighting, distance, poses each month to accurately assess adjustments needed. Notice energy levels and how clothing fits too.

Monitor Weight Weekly

Step on the scale at the same time each week to detect patterns over time. Remember that weight fluctuates daily and normal ranges are higher during menopause. Focus more on clothing fit, body measurements and how you feel. If the number motivates you, record it. If it discourages you, measurements may be better markers.

Record Symptoms

Tracking the duration, frequency and severity of menopausal symptoms helps identify correlations with potential dietary triggers. Hot flash patterns, migraine occurrences, bowel changes, yeast infections and urinary issues can all provide helpful insights. Rate symptoms daily from 1-10 to capture ups and downs.

Get Lab Work Done

Getting baseline lab tests for hormones, cholesterol levels, blood sugar, thyroid, CRP, nutrients like iron, vitamin D and B12 can reveal opportunities to tweak your diet. Ask for before/after comparisons to showcase improvements tied to nutritional changes over 3-6 months. Bring logs of your intake to identify any diet adjustments needed.

Take Monthly Photos

Comparisons of monthly progress pics reinforce positive changes more than the daily grind. Have someone else take front, back and side photos on the same day each month in the same outfits under consistent conditions. Review the college to identify changes needed or celebrate successes!

Measure Body Composition
Measurements with body tape and tools like the InBody machine showcase fat loss and muscle gain the scale doesn't show. Track total weight, body fat percentage, lean mass, visceral fat, body water percentage and skeletal muscle mass monthly under consistent conditions. This data reveals what dietary approaches and exercise regimens work best.

Track Nutrient Intake
Analysing your daily food logs in a tool like MyFitnessPal provides helpful metrics - calories, macronutrients, vitamins, minerals and more. Compare daily and weekly averages of protein, fibre, calcium, iron etc to recommended intake levels. Identify nutrient

gaps to address or excess sodium, sugar and saturated fats to limit.

Compare Inflammatory Markers

Getting blood tests done provides concrete markers of internal inflammation to compare over time. Key indicators include homocysteine, hs-CRP, Omega-3 Index and fasting insulin and glucose. Cholesterol panels also assess heart disease risk. Use diet tweaks and supplements to improve numbers.

Identify Food Sensitivities

Menopause can uncover food sensitivities leading to symptoms like GI issues, headaches, joint pain and sinus congestion. Track severity of symptoms daily for at least a week eating normally. Then eliminate suspect foods completely for 4 weeks, followed by measured reintroduction while tracking reactions. Common offenders include gluten, dairy, corn, soy and eggs.

Apps and journals

In addition to food logging apps, use apps like Flo to analyse your cycle and symptoms. Paper journals allow colouring, handwritten notes and designing pages precisely how you like. Try a combination so you always have one on hand.

Find Accountability Partners

Sharing your diet journey with a partner provides community, accountability and inspiration. Enlist gym friends, relatives undergoing similar transitions or online groups. Check in weekly on goals, wins, challenges where others can provide feedback and encouragement.

Celebrate Small Wins

Recognize little achievements along the way like eating 3 veggies at dinner for a week straight or having only water for 30 days. These milestones motivate you to keep going to reach bigger goals. Treat yourself to a massage, pedicure or fun outing - not food!

Tracking all aspects of your diet and symptoms provides visible proof of what's working...and what's not. Various logs, apps, community support and milestone rewards help motivate you through the menopause transition for better health. Be consistent tracking macros, symptoms, measurements and more to create your custom Menopause Manifesto plan.

Building a Sustainable and Enjoyable Menopause Diet Lifestyle

Here is a guide to building a sustainable and enjoyable menopause diet lifestyle:

The Key Principles

Sustainability - The changes you make need to be maintainable in the long run. Don't follow overly restrictive diets that are hard to stick to. Make gradual changes at a pace you can follow.

Nutrition - Focus your diet on whole, nutrient-dense foods that nourish your body and support hormonal balance. Minimise processed items.

Moderation - Allow yourself occasional treats that you really enjoy and savour them mindfully. Depriving yourself often backfires.

Self-Care - Be compassionate with yourself throughout the process. Honour when you need rest. Manage stress. Do activities you love.

Where to Begin

Start by keeping a 3-day food diary without changing anything. This highlights areas to improve. Are you eating enough protein and produce? Too many sugary treats? Not drinking enough water?

Develop SMART goals based on your biggest areas for improvement and your self-care needs. Perhaps cooking more plant-based home meals or a consistent bedtime.

Build Up Gradually

Pick 1-2 goals to focus on each week, not an overhaul. Maybe cooking two extra veggie sides per week or limit coffee to mornings only that week. Check off successes in a journal.

Over several months, these small changes create positive momentum to tackle bigger goals. New habits feel less intimidating and broken down.

Optimising Nutrition

Shift your plate balance to emphasise vegetables, high quality proteins, whole grains and healthy fats. Limit sweets and refined carbs. Stay hydrated with herbal tea and water.

Meal prep during high energy times so healthy options are grab'n-go when you're busy. Having salad ingredients washed and snacks portioned out makes better choices effortless.

Find Enjoyable Movement

Working out for sheer calorie burn can backfire by making exercise feel punitive. Instead explore enjoyable activities like dance, tennis, hiking or yoga for mental and physical renewal.

Recruiting friends makes fitness social and accountability partners keep you consistent. Switch things up when boredom hits.

Practise Mindful Eating

Savouring meals slowly without distractions allows you to tune into your true hunger and fullness signals. Check in - does this food actually make you feel good?

When an emotional craving hits, pause and ask where it's stemming from. Anxiety? Fatigue? Then address the root cause rather than mindlessly eating.

Staying consistent with sustainable changes empowers you to feel mentally sharp, energetic and healthy during menopause and beyond.

Conclusion

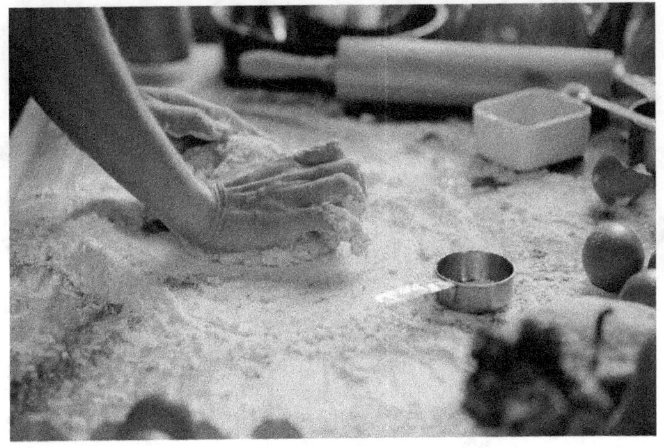

As you flip through these final pages, I hope you feel empowered, equipped and excited to nourish your body with incredible care during this transition and whatever lies ahead.

You now hold a trusty collection of delicious, nutritious recipes in the palm of your hand - ready to uplift your days with food that speaks to your soul.

May these meals give you the building blocks for blazing your unique health and happiness path forward - wherever it may lead. Remember - progress over perfection.

When challenges arrive, come back to these pages for comfort food to lift your spirit, reminders to toast all you've overcome, and inspiration to keep going.

Share these recipes with others who need them, so they too can feel held during the uncertainties that come with womanhood.

Trust that your ever-changing seasons are not to be endured, but provide chances for you to rediscover and celebrate your essence.

I hope cooking these recipes brings you moments of playfulness, nostalgia, intimacy and insight during the magical mystery tour to the wise, juicy crone waiting within. She can't wait to meet you.

Now, let's get cooking! This kitchen isn't going to clean itself...

With tremendous love and a sprinkle of parsley , Erin P. Walker.

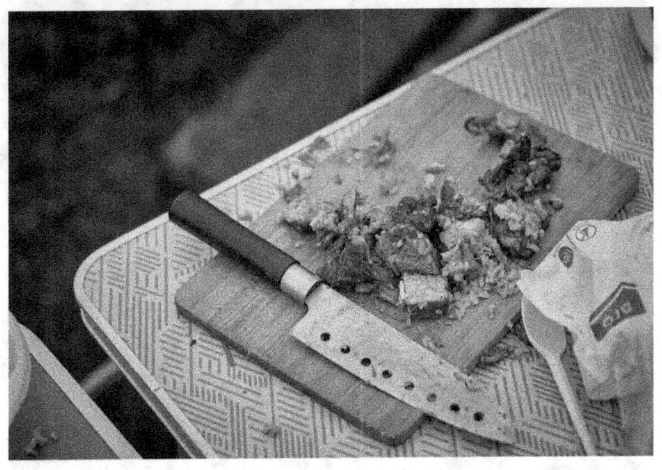

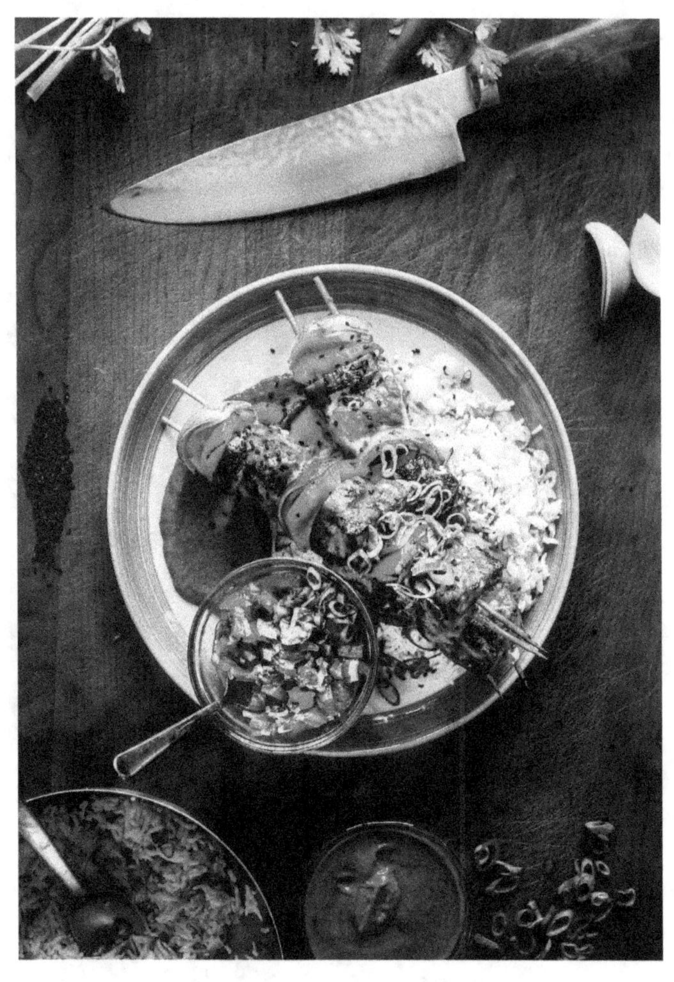

www.ingramcontent.com/pod-product-compliance
Lightning Source LLC
Chambersburg PA
CBHW070852260726
48661CB00004B/1374